ISBN: 978-1-7388833-5-6

"Your mental health is a priority.

Your happiness is essential.

Your self-care is a necessity." -

"Writing can be a powerful tool for healing and self-discovery. It allows us to give voice to our thoughts and emotions, and to explore our innermost selves with honesty and compassion

TABLE OF CONTENTS

HOW WRITING HELPS WITH MENTAL HEALTH

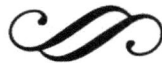

W riting can have a positive impact on mental health, particularly in helping individuals cope with stress, trauma, and unexpected life events. Expressive writing, which involves writing about thoughts and feelings that arise from a traumatic or stressful life experience, has been found to reduce stress, anxiety, and depression. It can also improve sleep, performance, and bring greater focus and clarity.

Expressive writing can be a useful tool for recording experiences and working through them.

Writing can also increase self-awareness, which is a significant link between writing and improved mental health. Writing can help individuals process difficult life events, gain clarity, and increase confidence. Writing can also clear the mind of worries, negative thoughts, or sources of pain.

A social psychologist James Pennebaker at the University of Texas studied the impact of writing on mental health in 1986 and found that "emotional writing" can have a positive effect on mental health. Since then, over 200 studies have reported similar findings. While it may seem counterintuitive that writing about negative experiences has a positive effect, some have posited that narrating the story can help individuals move beyond the experience.

While all writing can be good for mental health, there are particular types of writing, expressive writing, reflective writing, and creative writing. Writing is a powerful tool that can be used to support mental well-being and promote self-care.

Some people choose to write daily, while others may write less frequently. Journaling once a day, such as writing down five things that one is thankful for, can be a helpful practice for some individuals.

Rereading one's writing can also provide deeper insight into thoughts, feelings, behavior, and beliefs.

Writing for self-awareness can be a great place to start, and individuals can reflect on their feelings about a stressful event or a difficult work situation and consider what they have learned from it.

Research has shown that writing for just 20 minutes a day can have a positive effect on mental health. While all writing can be good for mental health, there are particular types of writing that are often mentioned in this context, including expressive writing, reflective writing, and creative writing. Ultimately, the frequency of writing should be determined by what makes the individual feel good and what works best for them. Writing authentically, with truth and openness, can be a helpful way to process emotions and experiences and improve mental health.

WHAT TYPES OF WRITING ARE MOST EFFECTIVE FOR IMPROVING MENTAL HEALTH

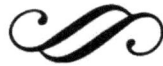

E xpressive writing, reflective writing, and creative writing are types of writing that are most effective for improving mental health. Expressive writing involves writing about thoughts and feelings related to a stressful life event, while reflective writing involves reflecting on past experiences and emotions.

Creative writing involves using imagination and literary devices like imagery and metaphor to convey meaning. Writing for self-awareness is also effective for improving mental health, as it can increase self-awareness and help individuals process difficult life events.

Guided journals, such as devotionals, mindfulness and meditation journals, mood journals, gratitude journals, self-esteem journals, wreck journals, and Bible and prayer journaling, can also be effective for improving mental health.

Ultimately, the most effective type of writing for improving mental health is the one that works best for the individual and allows them to express their thoughts and emotions authentically.

HOW CAN CREATIVE WRITING
HELP WITH MENTAL HEALTH

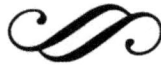

C reative writing can be a helpful tool for improving mental health. Creative writing, such as poetry, short stories, novellas, and novels, can encourage people to choose their words, metaphors, and images in a way that captures what they are trying to convey, leading to increased self-awareness and self-esteem.

Creative writing can also help individuals express their emotions and experiences to develop a deeper level of self-awareness, which can offer support towards becoming more resilient in the future. Writing about emotions and feelings that arise from a traumatic or stressful life experience, called expressive writing, can also help some people cope with the emotional fallout of such events.

WHAT ARE THE BENEFITS OF EXPRESSIVE WRITING FOR MENTAL HEALTH?

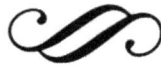

Expressive **Writing** is a type of writing that can be particularly effective for improving mental health. Expressive writing involves writing about thoughts and feelings related to a stressful life event, with the aim of helping emotionally process something difficult. Research shows that expressive writing can enhance self-awareness, ultimately decreasing depressive symptoms, anxious thoughts, and perceived stress.

Expressive writing can also result in a reduction in stress, anxiety, and depression, improve sleep and performance, and bring greater focus and clarity. Reflective writing and creative writing are other types of writing that can improve mental health.

Reflective Writing aims to give people a way to assess their experiences and emotions, while creative writing involves using imagination and literary devices to convey meaning. Ultimately, the most effective type of writing for improving mental health is the one that works best for the individual and allows them to express their thoughts and emotions authentically.

WRITING FOR
SELF-AWARENESS

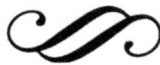

❧

Is a key component of good mental health. Self-awareness is the ability to recognize and understand one's own thoughts, feelings, and behaviors. Writing can help increase self-awareness by allowing individuals to reflect on their experiences, emotions, and beliefs.

Reflective writing, expressive writing, and creative writing are some types of writing that can improve self-awareness and mental health. Expressive writing involves writing about thoughts and feelings related to a stressful life event, while reflective writing involves reflecting on past experiences and emotions.

Creative writing involves using imagination and literary devices like imagery and metaphor to convey meaning. Increased self-awareness can lead to greater job satisfaction, better decision-making, and improved professional and personal relationships, all of which are indicators of good mental health.

Ultimately, writing can be a valuable tool for self-reflection, personal growth, and mental health.

WHAT ARE THE BEST JOURNALING TECHNIQUES FOR MENTAL HEALTH

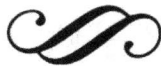

There are several journaling techniques that can be helpful for mental health. Stream-of-consciousness journaling is particularly helpful for individuals who are critical of themselves or have perfectionistic tendencies.

Expressive writing, reflective writing, and creative writing can all lead to increased self-awareness and improved mental health. Journaling can help individuals manage anxiety, reduce stress, and cope with depression.

Here are some specific journaling techniques that can be beneficial for mental health:

1. **Gratitude journaling:** Writing down five things that you are thankful for each day can help shift your focus to the positive aspects of your life.

2. **Future self-journaling:** Writing about your future self and the person you want to become can help you set goals and work towards them.

3. **Mindfulness journaling:** Writing about your thoughts and feelings in the present moment can help you become more aware of your emotions and improve your mood.

4. **Problem-solving journaling:** Writing about a problem you are facing and brainstorming solutions can help you gain clarity and reduce stress.

5. **Letter writing:** Writing a letter to someone, whether it be to express gratitude or to work through a conflict, can be a therapeutic way to process emotion.

Ultimately, the most important thing is to find a journaling technique that works for you and to write authentically with truth and openness.

WHAT ARE SOME OTHER FORMS OF JOURNALING THAT CAN BENEFIT MENTAL HEALTH

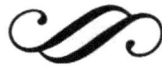

⤜⤝

There are many forms of journaling that can benefit mental health. Some examples include gratitude journaling, where individuals write down things they are thankful for, stream-of-consciousness journaling, where individuals write down their thoughts as they come to mind, and art journaling, where individuals use visual images and design to express themselves.

Prompts can also be helpful for individuals who are unsure of what to write about, and there are many resources available online. Journaling can help individuals manage symptoms of mental health challenges, create new life goals and healthy habits, and make sense of symptoms that are interfering in their lives.

Ultimately, the most effective form of journaling is the one that works best for the individual and allows them to express their thoughts and emotions authentically.

WHAT ARE SOME CREATIVE JOURNALING TECHNIQUES FOR MENTAL HEALTH

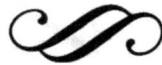

There are several creative journaling techniques that can benefit mental health. Creative journaling involves using different mediums such as art, music, or poetry to express thoughts and emotions.

Guided journals, such as devotionals, mindfulness and meditation journals, mood journals, gratitude journals, self-esteem journals, and wreck journals, can also be helpful.

Visual or art journaling can be a soothing, calming, healing, and stress-reducing activity, especially when individuals struggle with verbal self-expression.

Expressive writing through journaling can be a powerful way to process stress, trauma, and different emotions. Stream-of-consciousness journaling can be particularly helpful for individuals who are critical of themselves or have perfectionistic tendencies.

Ultimately, the most effective form of journaling is the one that works best for the individual and allows them to express their thoughts and emotions authentically.

WHAT ARE SOME CREATIVE JOURNALING TECHNIQUES FOR BEGINNERS

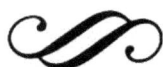

There are many creative journaling techniques that beginners can try.

Mind map journaling involves creating a visual representation of thoughts and ideas.

Story journaling involves writing fictional stories or personal narratives.

Dream journaling involves recording dreams and analyzing their meanings.

Music journaling involves writing about the emotions and memories that music evokes.

Art journaling involves incorporating art and drawing into journaling.

Photo journaling involves using photographs as prompts for writing.

Coloring journaling involves coloring pages and writing about the emotions and thoughts that arise.

Tracking journaling involves recording habits, moods, and goals.

Free writing journaling involves writing without any specific prompts or structure.

Mixed media journaling involves incorporating various forms of art and writing into journaling.

Ultimately, the best journaling technique is the one that works best for the individual and allows them to express their thoughts and emotions authentically.

CAN AUDIO-JOURNALING BE AS EFFECTIVE AS TRADITIONAL JOURNALING FOR MENTAL HEALTH?

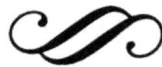

⌒𝒮𝒪⌒

Audio-journaling can be as effective as traditional journaling for mental health. Offers in-the-moment spontaneity that can help relieve anxiety and allows individuals to talk through their thoughts and emotions, which can be faster than writing them down.

Journaling, whether writing or audio recording, can support coping, reduce the impact of stressful events, and decrease mental distress.

Expressive, reflective, and creative writing can all lead to increased self-awareness, which is beneficial for mental health.

Ultimately, the most effective form of journaling is the one that works best for the individual and allows them to express their thoughts and emotions authentically.

HOW TO CHOOSE THE RIGHT JOURNALING METHOD

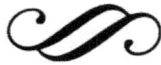

C hoosing the right journaling method depends on personal preferences and lifestyle. If an individual wants to record their day-to-day life, they may not need to spend thirty minutes journaling before bed. If an individual is sorting through difficult circumstances, they may want to pay attention to their dreams.

Stream-of-consciousness journaling is helpful for individuals who are critical of themselves or have perfectionistic tendencies. It is important to find a method that works for the individual and allows them to express their thoughts and emotions authentically.

Some tips for choosing the right journaling method that suits the individual, such as a physical diary or writing software, and finding what works best for the individual, whether it is typing or writing by hand.

Ultimately, the best journaling method is the one that the individual is excited about trying and that fits their lifestyle and preferences.

WHAT ARE SOME TIPS FOR MAKING JOURNALING A HABIT

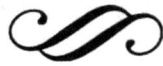

1. Choose a journaling method that suits your lifestyle and goals.
2. Start small and make it easy to stick to the habit. For example, write for just five minutes a day or choose a specific time of day to journal.
3. Remove distractions and find a quiet space to write.
4. Use prompts or guided journals to help get started.
5. Make journaling a part of your daily routine.
6. Track your progress and celebrate your successes.
7. Don't worry about doing it "right" or being perfect.
8. Remember that journaling is a personal practice, so find what works best for you and

HOW OFTEN SHOULD ONE WRITE TO SEE MENTAL HEALTH BENEFITS

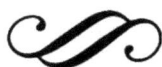

The frequency of writing required to see mental health benefits can vary depending on the individual and their goals. Some people may benefit from writing once a day, while others may find it helpful to write several times a day.

Expressive writing, reflective writing, and creative writing are all types of writing that can improve mental health. Writing for self-awareness is also a key component for good mental health. Journaling is a popular form of writing that can be done daily and has been shown to have positive effects on mental health.

Research has shown that writing for as little as 20 minutes a day can have a positive impact on mental health. Ultimately, the most effective frequency of writing for improving mental health is the one that works best for the individual and allows them to express their thoughts and emotions authentically.

WHAT ARE SOME WRITING PROMPTS FOR MENTAL HEALTH PURPOSES

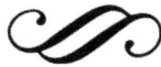

Here are some writing prompts for mental health purposes:

1. Reflect on a difficult life event and write about your thoughts and feelings related to it.
2. Make a list of things that make you happy, including both big and small things.
3. Write about a time when you overcame a challenge and what you learned from the experience.
4. Write about what you are grateful for in your life.
5. Write about your coping mechanisms and evaluate which ones are working for you.
6. Write a message to yourself for bad mental health days to remind yourself of happier times.

7. Write about a difficult work situation from the past year and consider what you have learned from it.
8. Write about your first coping mechanism that comes to mind when you are feeling stressed or anxious.
9. Write about what you would like to improve in your life and why.
10. Write about what's hardest for you in as many words as it takes.

These prompts can help you explore your thoughts and emotions and can be a helpful tool for self-reflection and personal growth.

WHAT ARE SOME TIPS FOR GETTING STARTED WITH WRITING FOR MENTAL HEALTH PURPOSES

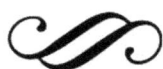

Here are some tips for getting started with writing for mental health purposes:

1. Choose a type of writing that resonates with you: There are different types of writing that can improve mental health, such as expressive writing, reflective writing, and creative writing. Choose the type of writing that you feel most comfortable with and that you think will be most effective for you.

2. Set aside time for writing: Schedule a regular time for writing, whether it's daily or weekly. This will help you establish a routine and make writing a habit.

3. Find a quiet and comfortable space: Choose a quiet and comfortable space where you can focus on your writing without distractions.

4. Write authentically: Write honestly and authentically, without worrying about what others might think. This will help you express your thoughts and emotions more effectively.

5. Use prompts: If you're not sure what to write about, use prompts to get started. Prompts can help you explore your thoughts and emotions more deeply.

6. Don't worry about grammar or spelling: Don't worry about grammar or spelling when you're writing for mental health purposes. The goal is to express your thoughts and emotions, not to write a perfect piece of literature.

7. Be patient: Writing for mental health purposes can take time, so be patient with yourself. Don't expect to see immediate results, but trust that writing can be a powerful tool for improving mental health over time.

The most important thing is to find a writing practice that works for you and that you enjoy.

HOW WRITING COMPARES
TO OTHER FORMS OF THERAPY
FOR MENTAL HEALTH

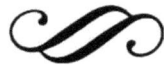

Writing is a powerful tool for mental health that can be done individually or guided by a mental health professional. Writing therapy can help individuals work through their thoughts and emotions, regulate their feelings, and even have physical benefits.

Writing therapy has many potential physical and psychological health benefits and can be used to treat people with many different conditions and stressful or traumatic experiences. Writing therapy can be compared to other therapies aimed at the same end, and it has been shown to be effective for different conditions and mental illnesses.

While writing therapy is a low-cost, easily accessible, and versatile form of therapy, true writing therapy would be conducted with the help of a licensed mental health professional.

www.ingramcontent.com/pod-product-compliance
Lightning Source LLC
Chambersburg PA
CBHW060601030426
42337CB00019B/3582